Confronting

Erectile

Dysfunction

Head-On

Symptoms, Causes & Treatment

Dr. Sheila Harrison

Disclaimer

This content serves to provide general information about the disease and aims to empower you to seek prompt medical assistance if necessary to prevent complications. It's essential to stress that this information is not a substitute for consulting a qualified physician. The field of medical science is continually evolving, and due to the dynamic nature of medical knowledge, we recommend seeking expert advice if you encounter any inconsistencies or intend to take action based on the information in this content. Never disregard professional medical guidance or delay treatment based on something you've read online, including this material, or from any other online source. Always remember that the internet cannot cure you; rather, healing comes through the guidance of medical professionals and the providence of God.

Table of Contents

Overview

The inability to maintain an erection during sexual activity is known as erectile dysfunction (ED). Not only can erectile dysfunction affect men, but if left untreated, it can severely damage a couple's ability to be intimate. Here are the opinions of specialists on the often disregarded matter of a man's health.

– to acknowledge, obtain medical attention, and solve the issue.

"It's a Man Thing: Below-the-Belt Conversation," an online conclave hosted by Boston Scientific, aimed to normalize the much-needed narrative surrounding ED.

- 10% of men have ED before the age of 40, while 50% of men over 40 suffer from it.

- Men with diabetes also have ED in 40% of cases.

- Obesity, alcoholism, and smoking are lifestyle variables that contribute to eating disorders.

- Before seeing the appropriate expert or doctor for ED, the majority of men opt to self-treat and rely on herbal remedies and supplements. It takes about four years to do this.

- Just one in three males with ED seek treatment.

- ED causes 20–30% of marriages to end in divorce.

These shocking numbers and facts were unveiled at the beginning of the Conclave to set the stage for specialists to identify the problem's likely roots, provide an understandable explanation of the situation, and address the physiological, psychological, sociological, and medical aspects of the problem.

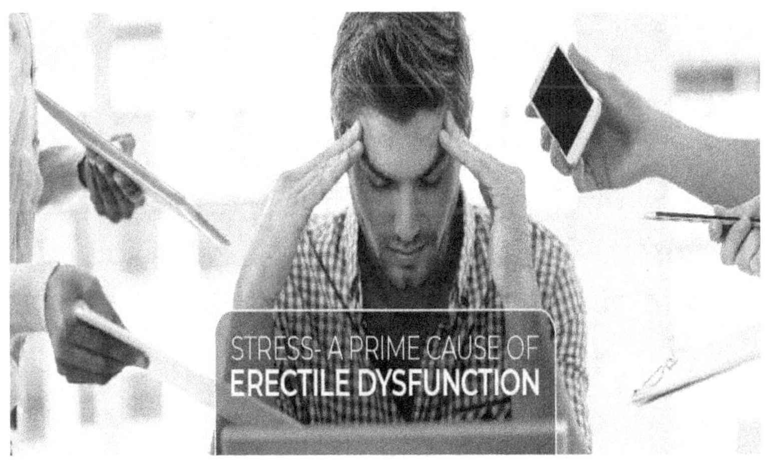

Section 1

What is Erectile Dysfunction (ED)?

Impotence, also referred to as erectile dysfunction (ED), is the inability for you or your partner to maintain an erection strong enough for engaging in sexual activity. Premature ejaculation or the inability to sustain an erection long enough for both people to engage in satisfying sexual activity can be the cause of ED. Failure to achieve an erection more than 50% of the time may indicate ED, albeit this is not always the case. Numerous things could be the cause, including stress, drinking, or damage or malformations to the penile blood vessels.

ED may be a chronic illness or a transient one. An estimated 10% of men experience ED over an extended period of time, typically affecting those over 40. According to a study conducted in the United States, roughly 52% of men suffer ED in some capacity, and the percentage of men who have ED overall rises from 5 to 15% between the ages of 40 and 70. Even though ED is more common in older adults, it can nonetheless affect young men.

ED can lead to a loss of intimacy between couples. However, most men do not get it treated due to a fear of embarrassment or because of societal stigmas towards ED. Treating ED should be normalized, as ED can also be a sign of other underlying medical conditions that are not detected.

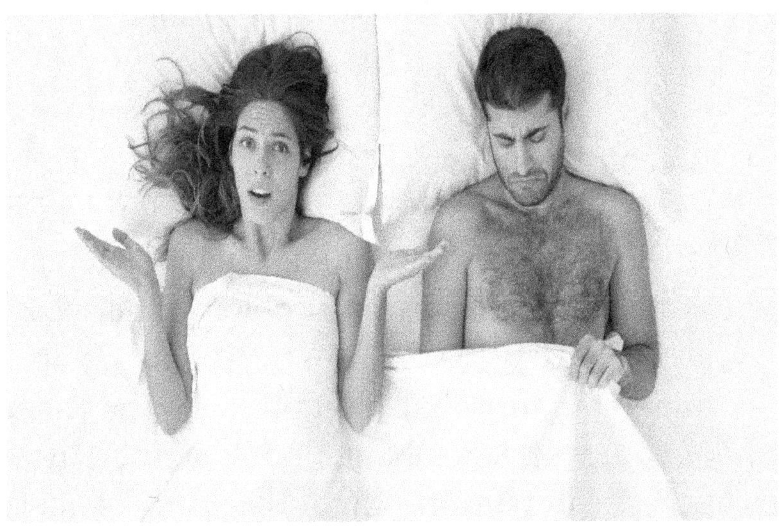

Section 2

Symptoms of Erectile Dysfunction (ED)

Understanding ED and its symptoms

The main symptoms of ED are the inability to get and keep an erection during sexual activities, as well as reduced libido, or sexual desire.

Erectile Dysfunction (ED) is just a descriptive term for a problem with the erection and not a label, a diagnosis or a stigma. Remember somebody who has no problem otherwise, can also have ED. We need to start by understanding that it's nothing to be ashamed of or worried about, and neither does it necessarily mean that there is something wrong.

A problem with erection, which is what it is, could happen in any young person, just because he was anxious or tense or misinformed or was trying to impress a new partner so could have ED due to performance anxiety. It could also happen in middle-aged men who again don't have a real problem, but they're stressed out, have work-related tension, work pressure, and come home very tired. And it could happen in older men who have an actual physical problem because of diabetes, hypertension, high cholesterol, smoking, all of which compromise the blood flow.

Some other symptoms may include having an erection outside of sexual activities, but not during; and an inability to maintain an erection during masturbation.

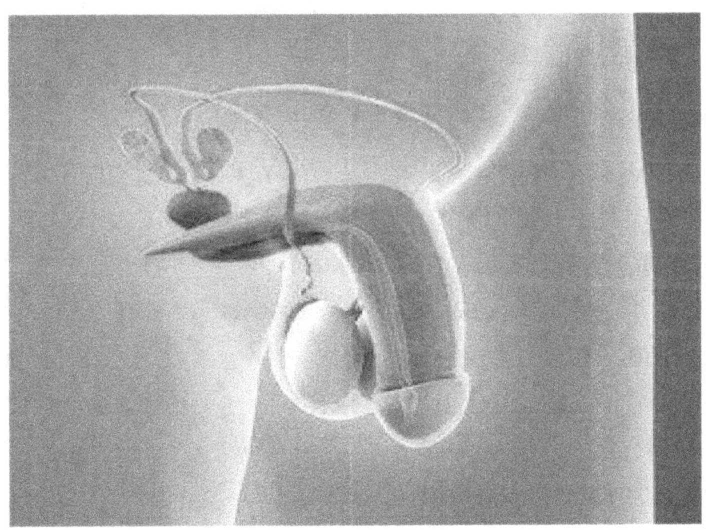

Section 3

Causes of Erectile Dysfunction (ED)

It takes patience and experience to find the right cause of ED. "It is a complex problem as it arises from the faulty interplay of the mind, the nerves, the arteries, the corporal sponge, the veins, and the influence of hormones. It can be both physiological or organic as well as psychological.

Listening to the patients to get to the root of the problem is key, which is going into the holes of what is happening in an individual's life. And that helps to make a proper diagnosis. The most important thing to do with patient is to spend time listening to their problems.

In most cases, the man's penis becomes the partner's or couple's phenomenon. Does the women come forward to help their partners work on ED so that the couple could lead a fuller life? When that happens you will later realize from their detailed history and findings, that there is a peculiar problem happening within the relationship or not which is affecting the erection.

ED Patients are also to know that, even if they have a problem with ED, that alone should send a signal of oneness with their partners hence try to solve this problem together with their partners. That's a lot of support, and such encouragement certainly helps the client.

There are a number of reasons that ED may occur, and it is not just because of psychological factors like stress or depression. These may include:

- Atherosclerosis (blocked blood vessels)
- Diabetes mellitus
- Hypertension
- Damage to the spinal cord
- Physical trauma
- Multiple sclerosis
- Alcoholism
- Frequent smoking
- Frequent Mustabation
- Low testosterone
- Hormone imbalance
- Side effects from certain medications
- Effects of surgery

- Drug abuse
- Parkinson's
- High cholesterol
- Work-related tension, work pressure
- Anxiety from misinformation - Trying to impress a New Partner
- Obesity increases the risks.

Having experienced any of these does not mean you will have ED, but they present a higher risk of getting it.

ED may be a sign of an underlying medical complication that may be present. A thorough diagnosis will usually be done to determine if this is true.

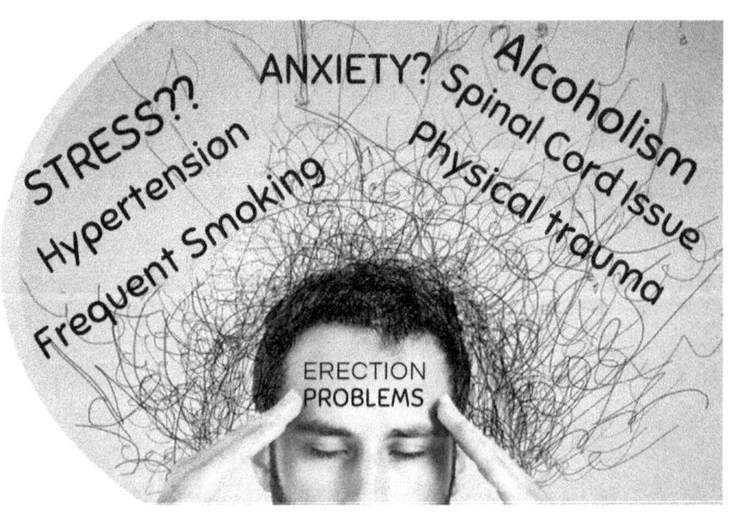

Section 4

Erectile Dysfunction Risk Factors

Obesity increases the risks

According to a study, about 30% of obese people who seek help in controlling weight indicate problems with sex drive, desire, performance, or all three. So, suppose a person desires to have a better sex life. In that case, the health goal should be to cut down on that extra weight and maintain an ideal weight because, all said and done, obesity is a barrier to enjoying the sexual experience thoroughly.

An individual is considered obese when the actual weight is 20% more than the ideal weight (as per the height). Obesity is one of the significant health challenges globally, especially in developed nations. It is the root cause of ill-health. Being overweight increases the risk of heart diseases, diabetes, hypertension, stroke, osteoarthritis, and cancers such as colon, pancreas, stomach, and breast. Unfortunately, obesity can be physically and psychologically restrictive, thus preventing intimacy, adversely impacting one's sex life.

Highlighting some lifestyle and medical issues in daily lives that are contributing to ED in terms of man capacity, let's not lose sight of the fact that Sex is best when you're at the peak of your health, then you have the greatest urge, the greatest energy, the greatest capability. As your general health diminishes, your sexual abilities decrease, even though that desire may be there. So the middle-aged executive who's overweight, not exercising, eating too much sugar, smoking 10 cigarettes a day is going to have a lifestyle-induced sexual problem.

Diabetes & Hypertension

It is imperative to realize that diabetes will affect the nerves, small blood vessels, the large blood vessels, the endocrine system, and predispose the men to erectile problems. Likewise with hypertension. Both hypertension and the medicines consumed to control hypertension could cause ED.

Stress Anxiety & Depression

Stress, anxiety, depression and mental health issues have aggravated during the pandemic and that adds to the intimacy woes. These contribute significantly and worsen the modern man's thing, while his capability goes down. What makes it worse is the acceptance of the fact that often people refuse to believe that they are depressed, anxious and stressed.

Stress plays a major role in an individual's relations causing a lot of relationship problems that go on to cause a lot of sexual problems

Section 5

Diagnosing Erectile Dysfunction (ED)

Your care professional may ask you a number of questions related to you or your partner's medical and sexual history. These can include questions of medications you or your partner are currently taking, medical conditions either of you may be having, and the level of satisfaction from sexual activity. It may be rather embarrassing to go into specifics, but this is the first step to helping remedy the situation. The International Index of Erectile Function (IIEF) is a type of questionnaire that may be used in the diagnosis to ask some of these questions.

A physical exam may also be conducted if the doctor feels it is needed. This can help identify the possible cause of the ED and help inform them of what follow up test is needed next, or if discussing a treatment plan might be required.

There are other tests that can be considered as well, such as blood tests and ultrasound imaging. These tests not only look into the cause of ED but may also shed light on underlying medical conditions that require medical attention. Your doctor will inform you if this is indeed the case. These are generally done only if your doctor has reasonable suspicion that there may be an underlying medical issue that warrants further investigation.

A psychological evaluation may be needed if the cause of ED is not due to a medical condition. Your doctor will carefully assess psychological factors that might be influencing performance. It may even be a case of performance anxiety, due to stress, low self-esteem or embarrassment. Your doctor may then decide if you will require counseling for follow up treatment.

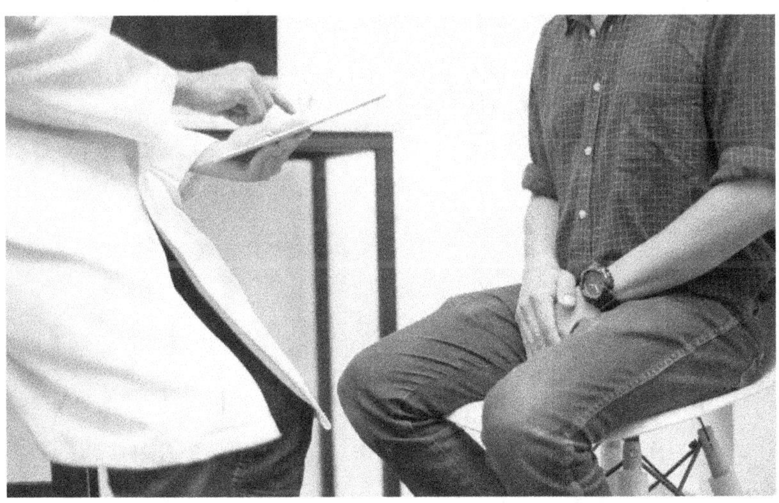

Section 6

Treating Erectile Dysfunction (ED)

Once a cause is ascertained, treatment can be very beneficial. "In organic ED, there is a need for long-term medications just like for any other disease arising from endothelial dysfunction like diabetes or cardiac illness. But in most cases, due to stigma and ignorance, patients refuse to seek help and prefer self-medication and Google-aided treatment that may do more harm than good.

But after a doctor has examined your medical and sexual history, they will decide on what the best treatment plan will be for you or your partner, with their associated benefits and risks.

Oral Medication

The pill is a double-edged sword. Those who are exploring self-medicating in such cases are losing out on the possibility of discovering why they are having the problem in the first place and solving the root cause of the problem. On the other hand, prescribed medicine work very well but the person is reluctant to take it because he is scared that it will harm him. I want to reassure men, and their partners, that using these medicines correctly are not dangerous. They do not damage the heart, kidneys or liver and can be taken long-term.

Medicines such as sildenafil (also known as Viagra), tadalafil (Cialis, Adcirca), and vardenafil (Levitra, Staxyn) are generally used to treat ED. They enhance the effects of nitric oxide, a natural chemical the body produces for relaxing the muscles in the penis, increasing blood flow to it and allowing you or your partner to get an erection.

In fact, Viagra (Sildenafil) was originally discovered in a Pfizer Lab while researching medicine for cardiac angina. Hence, it should not be taken by men who use medicine for angina (like Sorbitrate) as there will be a multiplying effect of the drug. Otherwise, it can safely be taken by men who are on antihypertensives or medicines for diabetes as long as they are otherwise physically fit for sex.

But because of that limitation, people have missed the point, thinking that it is bad for the heart, kidney and liver which is factually not true.

Taking these medications will still require sexual stimulation to produce an erection, and they are not aphrodisiacs that stimulate sexual desire. Ensure that you or your partner follow the prescription instructions at all times to prevent unwanted side effects.

Side effects may include flushing, nasal congestion, headaches, and indigestion. The dosage will be determined by your doctor, but always consult them if you frequently experience side effects, or if the medication has no effect at all. If you or your partner are having an erection that lasts more than 4 hours, immediately seek medical attention.

Oral medications are not to be taken if you are currently taking nitrate drugs used to treat chest pain, or angina, as it may result in hypotension (abnormally low blood pressure) that can be dangerous. You or your partner should also avoid taking these medicines if either of you has a heart-related condition.

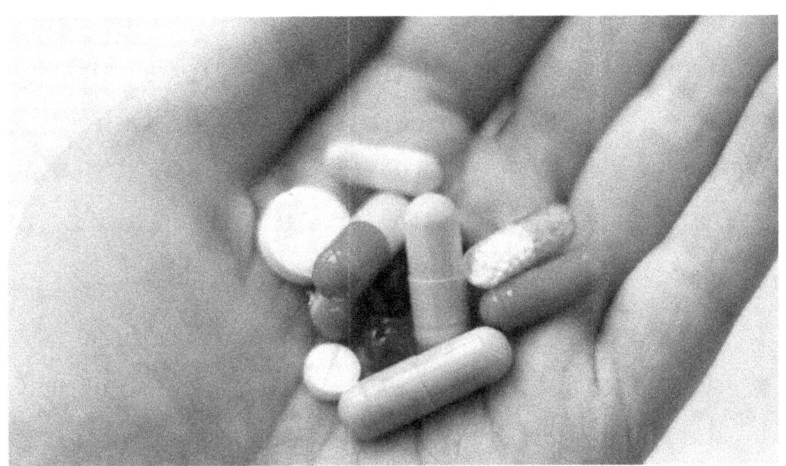

Non-oral Medications

In the event that you cannot take oral medications, there are other medications that may be prescribed to treat ED. One such medication is alprostadil, which can be prescribed in either a self-injection, a urethral suppository (a type of medicine that is inserted into the body, where it dissolves), or a topical cream.

The self-injection requires an injection of alprostadil (sometimes mixed with other medications) with a fine needle into the base or side of the penis. Each injection produces an erection that lasts no longer than an hour. As for the suppository, a tiny alprostadil suppository is placed into the penile urethra by means of a special device. The erection usually starts within 8 to 10 minutes and can last between 30 to 60 minutes.

However, the side effects of either method can be painful to you or your partner. Some side effects include minor bleeding from self-injection or in the urethra using the suppository; or even the formation of fibrous tissue inside the penis. Some with brain or blood-related conditions may even experience dizziness and high blood pressure.

Alprostadil topical creams are a less invasive method that simply requires the application of a medical cream to the penis. One study has found that the topical cream is a safer, painless way to treat ED, especially for those who cannot take oral medications.

Testosterone replacement therapy is also another consideration to treat ED. If the ED is caused by low levels of testosterone, then this will be recommended to treat it. It can help improve a man's energy, mood, bone density, as well as increase muscle mass and weight, and improve sexual desire. This is only recommended for men with low testosterone levels, as those with normal levels may experience side effects such as an enlargement of the prostate gland.

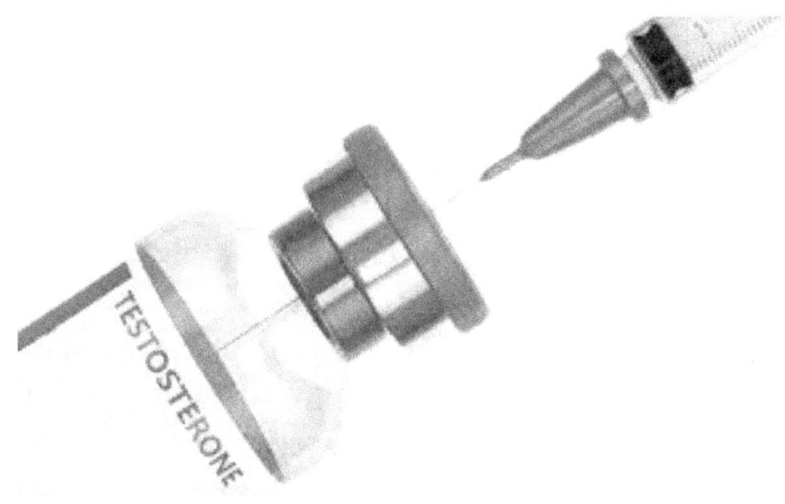

Mechanical Aids

This refers to medical devices that are approved for treating ED. One such device is a penis pump (vacuum constriction/erection device). Essentially, this device is a hollow tube on one end and a manually or battery-powered pump on the other. The device works by placing the penis into the tube, and then operating the pump to suck out the air inside the tube. This creates a vacuum within the tube that draws blood into the penis, causing an erection. Once done, a band (or tension ring) is slipped around the penis from the tube to maintain the erection before the pump is removed. The band can remain in place for up to 30 minutes; after sexual activity, you can remove the band.

While this is an effective way to treat ED, there are still complications that may arise from its use. For one, some complain that the penis pump is cumbersome and uncomfortable to use. Others find that their penis gets bruised when using it, and are put off by the fact that ejaculation is restricted because of the band.

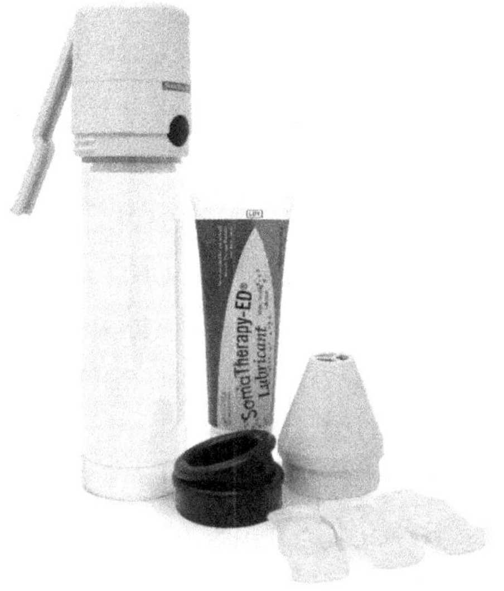

Penile Implants

This type of treatment involves surgery to insert devices into both sides of the penis, which allow you to manipulate them to produce an erection. The two most common types of implants are inflatable prostheses or malleable/semi-rigid prostheses.

The inflatable implant consists of a pump and two inflatable cylinders. The pump is usually located in the scrotum. By manipulating the pump, a saline solution is released into the cylinders (placed within the penis' erection chambers) and causes an erection. A deflation valve will remove the solution from these cylinders to deflate the penis after sexual activity.

The semi-rigid implant consists of bendable rods inserted into the penis' erection chambers, which can then be manipulated to produce an erection or reverse it.

Satisfaction ratings of men who received a penile implant are very favourable. Despite this, penile implants are considered a last resort measure where all other forms of treatment do not work. Side effects from the implants can be dangerous, as an infection is the most common cause for the implants to fail. Breakage can also be a major problem as well that will require immediate medical attention.

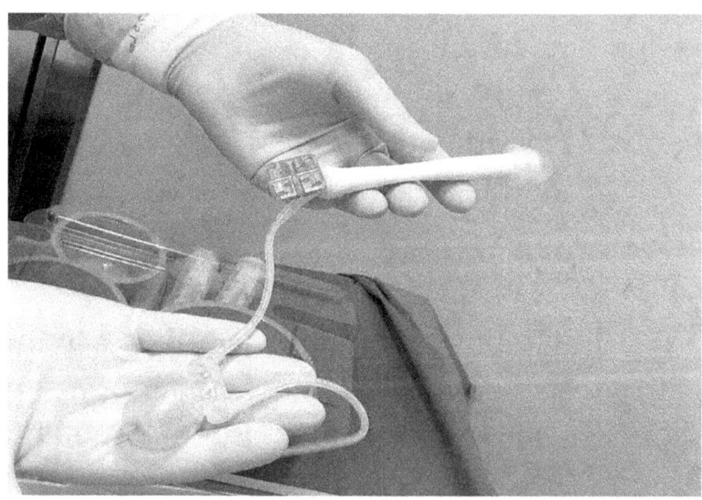

Psychological Counseling

Therapy is an effective treatment method for ED if it is caused by underlying emotional or psychological distress, and not due to a medical condition. A licensed counselor can help with relieving the emotional stress you may be experiencing, sometimes together with your partner to communicate how you feel with them.

It is perfectly fine if there is some embarrassment on the subject, but you or your partner should not keep hiding it or avoiding the problem. A lack of communication only serves to break down any measure of trust between couples and prolong the agony of having ED. Work through your anxieties, doubts and fears with the counsellor, and see what can be done to alleviate them. There are a wide array of therapy methods that will help you communicate your needs with your partner or to find new meaning in your relationship.

In the phycological counseling, most expert Follow a simple phenomenon — take into account a detailed sexual and relationship history. So that pretty much gives a wider view of what the cause can be.

- Is it an organic cause?
- Or is it something to be a psychological cause?
- Is it a social cause or it's absolutely a relationship problem which we are dealing with?"

When the causes are organic, a patient is referred to a physicians who specialize in that field, whether it's a cardiologist or an andrologist, and if it is a psychological cause, a patient is referred to psychiatrist or clinical sexologist to digs more into the detail to ascertain if the individual has primary ED or is it anxiety or depression or drug or alcohol or sometimes a partner's problem. "The partner must be suffering from some type of Vaginismus or desire disorder or depression, leading into ED. The psychiatrist or clinical sexologist try to find out if the couple has a relationship problem. If there's any, then in such patients, they look holistically on the triangle's three parts: the individual, the partner and the relationship," adds Dr Shyam.

ED has become an umbrella term for various issues that men may have in most cases. "It could be a libido problem, which means he doesn't feel the urge for sex, or he may have an arousal problem, he's not attracted to his partner, or he may have an erection problem, which again, maybe a problem with getting or sustaining an erection. And then sometimes, he may have a problem with early orgasm or premature ejaculation. Each of these conditions have different causes and treatments but all are clubbed under the umbrella term ED, which is not the case.

ED is one of the most common complaints cases at most health centers yet most patients are quite reluctant to speak about it, but the comfort has increased over decade as this trend is gradually changing. Most patients have psychogenic ED, which usually results from false perceptions or failures in intimacy due to anxiety and poor sexual education. Typically counseling and a few medications to instill confidence are all we need for many patients. In patients with psychogenic ED, the problem is curable if intervention happens in time. After a couple of weeks or months, most patients won't need any therapy.

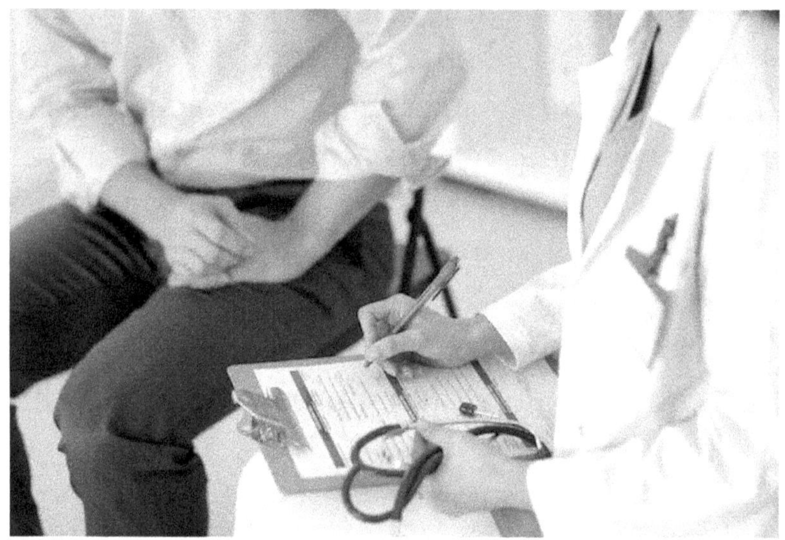

Section 7

Preventing Erectile Dysfunction (ED)

While some cases of ED are unavoidable, there are ways that you can prevent ED from ever happening to you. Most of these involve making important lifestyle changes that will improve your well-being. These include:

- Having a healthy, well-balanced diet
- Quit smoking
- Regular exercise
- Avoid drug abuse
- Reduce alcohol intake
- Follow your medicine schedule
- Communicate your feelings with your partner

Do not immediately take stock in claims of alternative medicine being able to cure ED, as many alternative cures may be based on pure speculation. Without proper clinical trials to prove their efficacy, taking these cures may be hazardous to your health. Always consult a licensed medical professional if you are considering taking any form of supplement.

An open conversation about sexual activity with your partner and your doctor is an important first step to combating ED.

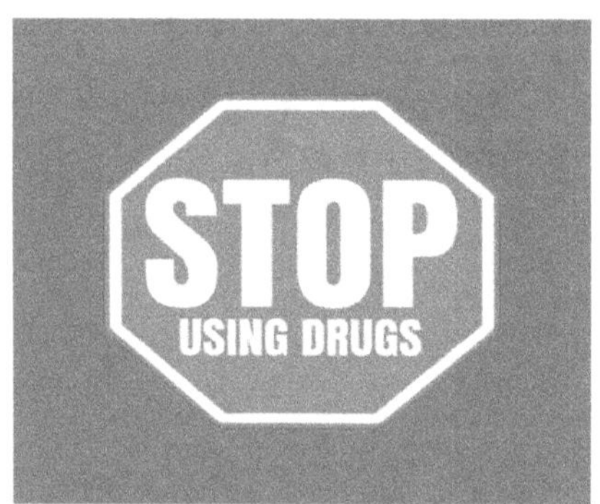

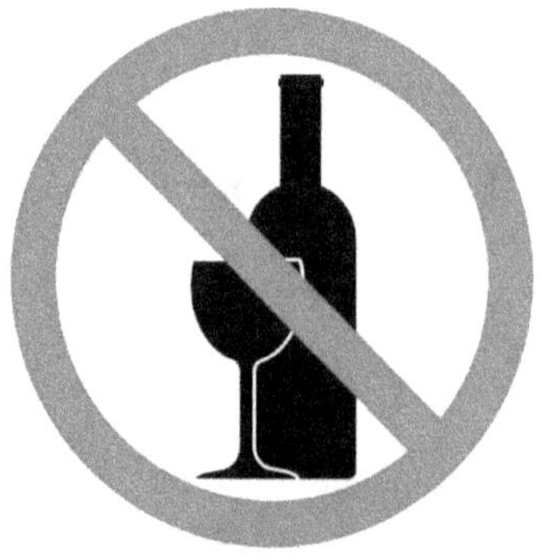

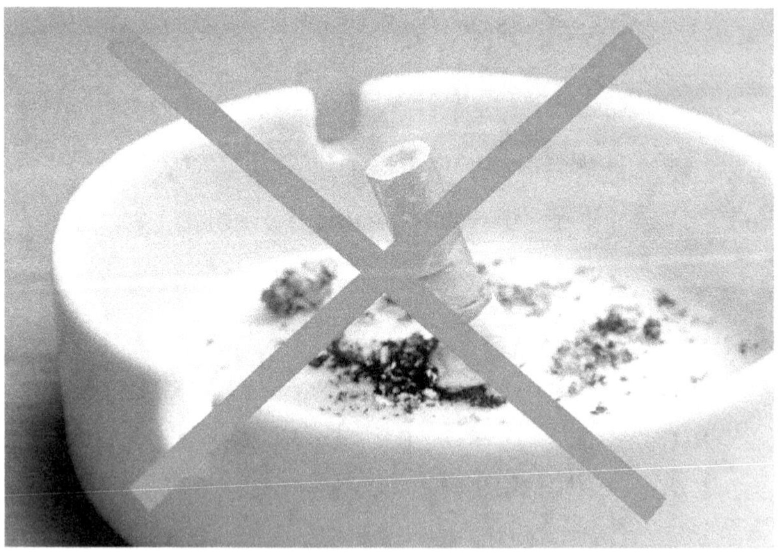